FRUITS FOR TWO
The Ultimate Guide For Expectant Mothers

Marya G. Qualls

Copyright Page

Fruits for Two

INTRODUCTION

Accommodating another existence

Being a mother is an incredible journey, composed of a sequence of joys, trust, and deep transformations. Everything changes for a woman when she discovers she is expecting a child. As she grows, her goals shift, and she feels compelled to really concentrate on and protect others. In "fruits for twos," Marya G. Qualls explores how important natural goods may be throughout this incredible journey. She provides pregnant women with a guide to the vitamins, flavors, and medicinal benefits that come with nature's greatest gifts.

Pregnancy is the best time to be happy, yet it can also be a stressful and unpredictable time. A pregnant woman may have several questions, such as what to eat and what to avoid, as well as how to ensure that she and the child are healthy. The modern world usually confuses matters by providing an overwhelming amount of nutrition advice and data that does not check up. Marya G. Qualls responds directly and clearly to this disaster: the power of fruit.

Exploring nutritional requirements

One of the most pressing issues for pregnant women is ensuring that they get enough nutrition to support the growth of their children. Pregnancy significantly increases a woman's nutritional requirements, and inadvertently consuming major nutrients and minerals might cause problems. However, navigating the food maze may be challenging. What is protected? What is useful? How can one ensure that a successful feast serves these more important needs without succumbing to pressure?

In "fruits for twos," Qualls discusses this very issue. She demystifies the nutritional requirements of pregnancy, demonstrating that organic goods are a pleasant, enjoyable, and very beneficial component of a healthy prenatal diet. Organic foods are high in nutrients, easy to prepare, and generally delicious, making them the perfect companion for expectant mothers looking to care for themselves and their children.

Sorcery of fruits: Nature's Vitamin Powerhouses

Fruits are nature's multivitamins, packed with important nutrients that are required throughout pregnancy. They are high in nutrients like C and A, minerals like potassium and folate, and cell Antioxidantss that benefit both the mother and the child's health. Qualls takes readers on a journey through the vibrant world of organic goods, concentrating on the unique benefits each one provides during pregnancy.

Consider the vital orange. Oranges are high in Vitamin c acid, which helps to strengthen the immune system, aid in iron absorption, and maintain healthy skin. Bananas, with their high potassium content, may help manage circulatory strain and avoid pregnancy-related enlargement. Berries are high in nutrients and promote the immune system. They also provide a sweet, satisfying bite that may help curb sugar cravings.

Accounts of Eager Mothers: Genuine Motivations

Qualls' tale is filled with examples of actually pregnant women who have recognized the power of plants. These testimonies are not only inspiring; they are also rational and helpful, providing readers with a quick glimpse into the lives of women who have overcome the difficulties of pregnancy with the help of nature's resources.

Consider the case of Sarah, who suffered from a severe morning illness throughout her most memorable trimester. Conventional medications offered little help, but she found consolation in the subtle causticity and cooling flavor of watermelon. Aside from the fact that it relieved her illness, its high water content kept her hydrated—an important factor throughout pregnancy.

Consider Emma, who had prenatal diabetes and anticipated regulating her eating habits to keep her glucose levels normal. She discovered that apples, with their high fiber content, helped manage her glucose and provided a delicious, satisfying bite that kept her energy levels stable throughout the day.

Evidence-Based Experiences: The Science Behind the Advantages

Qualls does not rely just on private evidence; she delves into the facts behind why vegetables are particularly beneficial during pregnancy. She explores how Fruit Vitamins enhance child development, from brain development to bone structure, and how they might help alleviate common pregnancy side symptoms such as congestion, expanding, and tiredness.

For example, folate, found in abundance in oranges, bananas, and avocados, is important for the formation of the brain tube, which forms the child's cerebrum and spinal cord. Sufficient folate intake reduces the chance of brain tube absconds, making it an important Vitamin throughout the third trimester. Essentially, fiber included in foods such as apples and pears may help manage obstruction, which is a typical problem among pregnant women.

Useful Exhortation: Integrating fruits into Your Eating Routine.

"Fruits for twos" is more than just a hypothetical study; it is a practical guide packed with advice and techniques for incorporating organic items into a daily diet. Qualls provides simple-to-follow recipes, snack ideas, and supper designs that make it easier for expectant women to enjoy the benefits of organic food without feeling concerned.

She suggests starting the day with a Vitamin-rich drink and combining food sources such as bananas, berries, and spinach for a delicious and energizing breakfast. For lunch, a fantastic Fruit salad might provide a delicious and Vitamin-rich meal. Furthermore, for those with midday desires, a simple bunch of grapes or a chopped apple with almond spread may be a delicious and nutritious meal.

Tending to the usual concerns: security and assortment.

One common worry among pregnant women is the safety of certain food types, and vegetables are no exception. Qualls addresses these difficulties fully, providing clear guidelines for which natural items are safe to ingest, which should be consumed with caution, and which should be avoided.

She emphasizes the need to thoroughly wash vegetables to remove any synthetic compounds or toxins, and she recommends adopting natural choices wherever possible. She also emphasizes the benefits of variety, encouraging pregnant women to consume a variety of foods to ensure they get a diverse range of nutrients.

Close to home and mental benefits: natural goods for the spirit

While the advantages of fruits are obvious, Qualls also explores their psychological and emotional effects. Pregnancy may be a time of elevated emotions and stress, and the simple act of consuming a Fruit can provide a moment of calm and happiness.

Organic items, with their clear tones, beautiful surfaces, and sweet flavors, may improve one's mood and create a feeling of comfort. Qualls urges pregnant women to take advantage of these moments and plan their days around consuming fruits that bring them pleasure and relaxation. Whether it's eating berries while reading a favorite book or sharing a Fruit platter with friends and family, these little acts of self-care may have a significant impact on mental health.

Beyond Sustenance: A comprehensive methodology

"Fruits for twos" is more than just a nutrition guide; it is a comprehensive approach to pregnancy health. She encourages pregnant women to perceive fruits as both nourishment and part of a larger lifestyle that values health, happiness, and relationships.

She discusses the social relevance of organic goods, their involvement in global traditions and customs, and their ability to unify people. Adding veggies to their daily routines allows expectant moms to connect with nature, their bodies, and their networks in meaningful ways.

The Creator's Excursion: A Unique Interaction

Marya G. Qualls writes with knowledge and compassion gleaned from her experience. As a mother herself, she understands the joys and difficulties of pregnancy, and her experience infuses her writing with realism and compassion.

Qualls discusses her own experiences, from the aspirations she had to the natural things that offered her pleasure and nourishment throughout her pregnancy. Her personal connection to the subject adds depth and attractiveness to her tale, bringing "fruits for twos" closer to home and attracting readers.

Encouragement to Embrace the Excursion.
As you open the pages of "fruits for twos," you will be approached with a sense of enthusiasm and joy to embark on the pregnant journey. Qualls' writing is more than just informative; it is persuasive and powerful, allowing pregnant mothers to confide in facts about their bodies and the outside world.

This book is a celebration of life's finest moments, an homage to the little pleasures that may have a tremendous impact. It exemplifies how, despite the complexities and demands of pregnancy, there is beauty and happiness to be found in the daily display of caring for oneself and one's child.

Conclusion: A sweet start.

"Fruits for twos" is more than just a book; it's a pregnancy resource. It contains useful ideas, logical experiences, and meaningful anecdotes that will inspire and assist pregnant women on a daily basis.

Allow Marya G. Qualls to guide you through this ever-changing journey with her wisdom and love. Accept the pleasantness of fruits, the vitality they provide, and the joy they provide. In the simple act of engaging in nature's richness, you will discover a source of solidarity, peace, and companionship that will benefit your pregnancy and beyond.

In this fashion, take a bite, enjoy the taste, and let the adventure begin. "fruits for twos" is here to take care of your body, support your brain, and share in the incredible experience of bringing new life into the world.

Chapter 1

The significance of a healthy diet during pregnancy

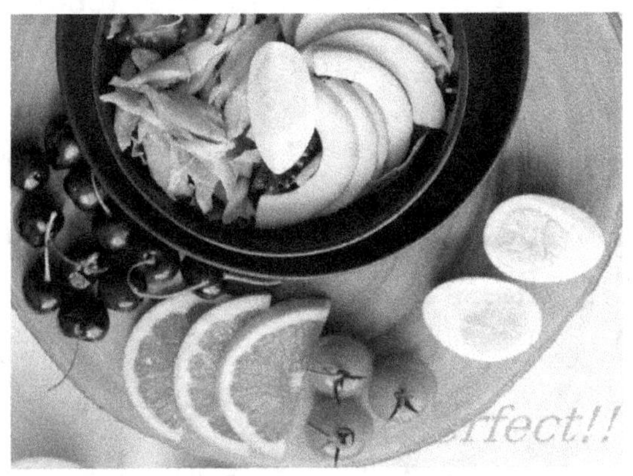

Yes, eating a balanced diet during pregnancy is very vital for both the mother and the baby.

A well-balanced diet supplies and furnishes the mother with key nutrients such as folic acid, iron, calcium, and protein, all of which are necessary for the baby's growth. High blood pressure and gestational diabetes are two more issues that it helps to prevent and treat. A healthy diet promotes development of the infant.

A good diet helps the baby develop, lowers the chance of birth defects, and improves general well-being for both mother and child. Quall discusses her experience with the necessity of a healthy diet during pregnancy.

Quall, a young pregnant woman, resided in the beautiful village of Meadowbrook, surrounded by rolling hills and lush foliage. Quall was cheerful when she figured out she was pregnant, however she immediately discovered that this exquisite experience required cautious consideration regarding her wellbeing and food.

As she began her pregnancy adventure, Quall sought advice from Dr. Morgan, a knowledgeable and kind obstetrician in town.

Dr. Morgan highlighted the necessity of a balanced diet during pregnancy, noting that it was more than simply gratifying desires; it was also about fueling her body and supporting her baby's growth and development.With Dr.

Morgan's advice in mind, Quall started to emphasize nutrient-rich foods in her daily diet. She ate enough fruits, veggies, whole grains, and lean meats, ensuring she got enough folic acid, iron, calcium, and protein.

As the weeks went by, Quall turned out to be more mindful of the decency of her great dietary patterns. She had more prominent energy, felt less depleted, and had less pregnancy-related side effects. Dr. Morgan gave her certainty that her commitment to eating great will help her as well as give serious areas of strength for her youngster's wellbeing.

One day, while browsing around the local market, Quall came upon Mrs. Thompson, an old lady noted for her knowledge and compassion. Mrs. Thompson discussed her personal maternity experiences and stressed the importance of eating nutritious meals while pregnant.

She described how, decades ago, access to dietary advice during pregnancy was restricted, and many women suffered from nutritional inadequacies that resulted in problems during delivery. Mrs. Thompson reminded Quall to appreciate the opportunity to make educated dietary choices and to prioritize her pregnant child's health.

Mrs. Thompson's comments powered Quall's craving to carry on with a better way of life. She attempted various recipes, went to pre-birth nourishment courses, and encircled herself with a steady organization of other hopeful ladies.

As the months passed, Quall's determination took care of in manners she would never have anticipated. Her kid developed hearty and sound in the belly, achieving every achievement with energy and enthusiasm. At the point when the opportunity arrived for Quall to conceive an offspring, she did as such with certainty, realizing that she had done all she could to give her child the best conceivable beginning throughout everyday life.

Quall's experience instructed her that a nutritious eating regimen during pregnancy is something beyond sustenance; it shows her adoration and obligation to her kid, a gift that will influence their lives until the end of time.

The Advantages of Including Fruits in a Pregnancy Diet.

Quall perceived the meaning of eating great all through her pregnancy and really tried to remember a lot of fruits for her everyday dinners. Each day, she would begin her day with a lovely Fruit salad, which included new berries, cuts of succulent melon, and bits of tasty pineapple.

Quall was happy with every feast, realizing that she was filling her body and empowering her child's advancement with the normal integrity of fruits. As the days went by, she began to find the uncommon benefits of remembering fruits for her eating regimen all through her pregnancy.

Her expanded energy level was quite possibly of the most perceptible improvement. In spite of the obligations of pregnancy, Quall felt more empowered and revived over the course of the day, attributable to the fruits she ate. Whether it was the zesty taste of citrus fruits or the fresh pleasantness of apples, each Fruit she ate appeared to fill her with new energy.

Fruits gave her energy, however they likewise freed some from the typical inconveniences of pregnancy. The fiber-rich nature of fruits assisted with keeping up with routine ness in her gastrointestinal system, easing the aggravation of swelling and stoppage that frequently impacted pregnant ladies.

Quall felt comfort in realizing that simply participating in nature's extravagance would alleviate her distresses and advance ideal stomach wellbeing.

Moreover, how much nutrients and minerals contained in fruits contributed fundamentally to Quall's overall wellbeing all through her pregnancy.

Citrus fruits incorporate Vitamin c acid, which reinforces her invulnerable framework, shields her from occasional diseases, and gives a sound climate to her creating kid.

In the meantime, the potassium-rich bananas assisted control her blood with constraining, bringing down the opportunity of issues and supporting a smooth pregnancy.

As Quall kept on featuring fruits in her eating routine, she was flabbergasted at the many benefits they gave all through her pregnancy. fruits shaped a significant piece of her pre-birth nourishment program, giving supporting Vitamins as well as splendid eruptions of taste.

As time passes, Quall feels a mind-boggling sensation of appreciation for the normal wealth of foods grown from the ground, significant impact they had on her wellbeing and the prosperity of her pregnant youngster.

As she restlessly looked for her youngster's introduction to the world, she set out to keep valuing the force of products of the soil significant benefits they gave all through her pregnancy.

A quick outline of the advantages of including fruits in a pregnancy diet.

1. Nutrient-dense: Fruits include critical vitamins, minerals, and antioxidants such as vitamin C, potassium, folate, and fiber, all of which promote general health and development during pregnancy.

2. Promotes Digestive Health: Fruits' fiber content helps avoid constipation, which is common during pregnancy, and promotes good digestion.

3. Boosts Immunity: Fruits include vitamin C, which helps the mother and baby fight infections and diseases.

4. Provides Energy: The natural sugars found in fruits offer a rapid and nutritious source of energy, reducing weariness and supporting the mother's increased energy requirements throughout pregnancy.

5. Aids in Hydration: Many fruits contain a lot of water, which helps keep the mother hydrated, which is particularly essential during pregnancy when fluid requirements are increased.

6. Promotes Fetal Development: Folate-rich fruits, such as oranges and strawberries, help to avoid neural tube abnormalities and promote appropriate fetal brain and spinal cord development.

7. Regulates Blood Pressure: Fruits high in potassium, like bananas and avocados, help to manage blood pressure and reduce the risk of problems like preeclampsia.

8. Helps with Weight Gain: Because fruits are low in calories and fat yet abundant in critical nutrients, they are an excellent option for regulating weight gain during pregnancy.

9. Provides Natural Sweetness: Fruits may fulfill sweet cravings in a healthier manner than commercial desserts or snacks, therefore contributing to a well-balanced diet.

10. Improves Skin Health: Fruits contain antioxidants, which help to maintain healthy skin, reduce the risk of stretch marks, and promote a bright complexion throughout pregnancy.Incorporating a variety of fruits into a pregnancy diet may improve the health and well-being of both the mother and the baby.

Chapter 2

Nutritious Requirements for Expectant Mothers

As Quall's pregnancy advanced, she came to comprehend that it was so pivotal to deal with her dietary prerequisites to guarantee both a sound pregnancy and the most ideal development for her unborn kid.

Through her own review and the counsel of Dr. Morgan, Quall found the exact Vitamins that were fundamental at this remarkable time of her life.

At the first spot on the list was folate, a B nutrient that is basic for early stage development. Quall ensured her child approached a sound eating routine that remembered food varieties high for folate, for example, citrus fruits, mixed greens, and strengthened grains, to keep away from brain tube irregularities and advance solid cerebrum and spinal rope improvement.

Quall additionally committed exceptional regard for iron, another fundamental nutrient. Her prerequisite for iron developed all through pregnancy, alongside her blood volume.

Lean meats, vegetables, and strengthened cereals are among the iron-rich things she added to her eating routine to keep away from pallor and ensure her child was getting sufficient oxygen. Quall likewise put an extraordinary worth on calcium.

She knew that calcium was fundamental for the development of bones and the appropriate activity of nerves, so she made a point to get her suggested day to day admission of calcium from dairy items, tofu, and mixed greens.

Quall also understood the significance of protein for the growth and development of her child. She made sure to provide her child with the building blocks for healthy cells Quall additionally grasped the meaning of protein for the development and improvement of her youngster.

She made a point to furnish her kid with the structure blocks for sound cells and tissues by consuming a scope of protein sources, including fish, chicken, eggs, lentils, and nuts.

Quall focused on including omega-3 unsaturated fats as an extra part in her eating regimen. She knew that her child's development of the mind and eyes relied upon these essential lipids. Quall ate pecans, chia seeds, and greasy fish like salmon to build her utilization of omega-3s.

Quall took comfort in the information that she was giving sound, Vitamining thick feasts for both herself and her unborn youngster as she dealt with her dietary requests during her pregnancy. She felt engaged with each feast, realizing that she was making way for her youngster's drawn out wellbeing and prosperity.

Through her experience, Quall discovered that pregnancy was more than basically wants and distress

it was likewise a chance to give taking care of oneself a high need and pursue choices that would influence her family's future.

Outfitted with intelligence and resolve, Quall acknowledged the dietary necessities of her pregnancy with appreciation and beauty, relishing the entire mind boggling experience tissues by consuming a range of protein sources, including fish, chicken, eggs, lentils, and nuts.

Quall concentrated on including omega-3 fatty acids as an additional component in her diet. She was aware that her baby's growth of the brain and eyes depended on these vital lipids. Quall ate walnuts, chia seeds, and fatty seafood like salmon to increase her consumption of omega-3s.

Here are some key nutrients that play a crucial role during pregnancy

1. Folate (Folic Acid): Folate is essential for proper neural tube formation in the early stages of pregnancy, which prevents birth defects like spina bifida. Pregnant women should aim to consume 600-800 micrograms of folic acid daily, primarily through foods such as leafy greens, citrus fruits, fortified cereals, and legumes.

2. Iron: Iron is necessary for the production of red blood cells, which transport oxygen throughout the body. During pregnancy, a woman's blood volume increases, and her iron needs rise as well. Iron-rich foods like lean meats, poultry, fish, fortified cereals, beans, and dark leafy greens should be included in the diet to prevent iron-deficiency anemia.

3. Calcium: Calcium is urgent for the improvement of the child's bones and teeth, as well with respect to keeping up with the mother's bone wellbeing. Pregnant women should aim for 1,000 milligrams of calcium per day, which can be obtained from dairy products, fortified plant-based milk, tofu, almonds, and leafy greens.

4. Protein: Protein is essential for the growth and development of the baby's cells and tissues. Pregnant women should consume about 71 grams of protein per day, sourced from lean meats, poultry, fish, eggs, dairy products, legumes, nuts, and seeds.

5. Omega-3 Fatty Acids: Omega-3 fatty acids, particularly DHA (docosahexaenoic acid), are critical for the development of the baby's brain and eyes. Pregnant women should include sources of omega-3s in their diet, such as fatty fish (salmon, sardines), flaxseeds, chia seeds, walnuts, and fortified foods.

6. Iodine: Iodine is important for thyroid function and the development of the baby's brain and nervous system. Pregnant women should consume 220 micrograms of iodine per day, which can be obtained from iodized salt, seafood, dairy products, and seaweed.

7. Vitamin D: Vitamin D is necessary for calcium absorption and bone health. Pregnant women should aim for 600 IU (International Units) of vitamin D per day, obtained from sources such as fortified foods, fatty fish, egg yolks, and exposure to sunlight.

8. Vitamin C: Vitamin C is important for immune function and the absorption of iron. Pregnant women should consume plenty of fruits and vegetables rich in vitamin C, such as citrus fruits, strawberries, kiwi, bell peppers, and broccoli.

Meeting these nutritional needs through a varied and balanced diet is essential for supporting the health and well-being of both the mother and the developing baby during pregnancy.

In some cases, prenatal Vitamins may be recommended to ensure adequate intake of certain nutrients. It's important for pregnant women to consult with their healthcare provider to address any specific dietary concerns or requirements.

Overview of Essential Nutrients

1. Protein: Protein is essential for building and repairing tissues, as well as for making enzymes, hormones, and other body chemicals. Good sources of protein include meat, poultry, fish, eggs, dairy products, legumes, nuts, and seeds.

2. Carbohydrates: Carbohydrates are the main fuel for the body. They are found in foods like grains, fruits, vegetables, and legumes. Whole grains, fruits, and vegetables also provide fiber, which aids in digestion and helps maintain bowel health.

3. Fats: Fats are necessary for absorbing certain vitamins, protecting organs, and providing energy. Healthy sources of fats include avocados, nuts, seeds, olive oil, fatty fish (like salmon and sardines), and dairy products.

4.   Vitamins: Vitamins are essential micronutrients that play various roles in the body, including supporting immune function, metabolism, and overall health. Examples include vitamin A (found in liver, sweet potatoes, and carrots), vitamin C (found in citrus fruits and bell peppers), vitamin D (found in fatty fish and fortified foods), and vitamin K (found in leafy greens).

5.   Minerals: Minerals are necessary for maintaining proper bodily functions, such as bone health, nerve function, and fluid balance. Important minerals include calcium (found in dairy products and leafy greens), iron (found in meat, beans, and fortified cereals), potassium (found in bananas, potatoes, and spinach), and magnesium (found in nuts, seeds, and whole grains).

6. Water: Water is essential for hydration and helps regulate body temperature, transport nutrients, and remove waste products from the body. It's important to drink an adequate amount of water each day to maintain optimal health.

7. Omega-3 Fatty Acids: Omega-3 fatty acids are a type of polyunsaturated fat that are important for heart health, brain function, and reducing inflammation. They are found in fatty fish (such as salmon, mackerel, and trout), flaxseeds, chia seeds, walnuts, and algae Vitamins.

8. Fiber: Fiber is a type of carbohydrate that the body cannot digest. It helps promote digestive health, regulate blood sugar levels, and lower cholesterol. Fruits, vegetables, whole grains, beans, and legumes are excellent sources of fiber.

Ensuring a balanced diet that includes a variety of nutrient-rich foods is essential for meeting the body's needs and maintaining overall health and well-being.

If you have specific dietary concerns or requirements, it's always best to consult with a healthcare provider or registered dietitian for personalized guidance.

Role of Fruits in Meeting Nutritional Requirements

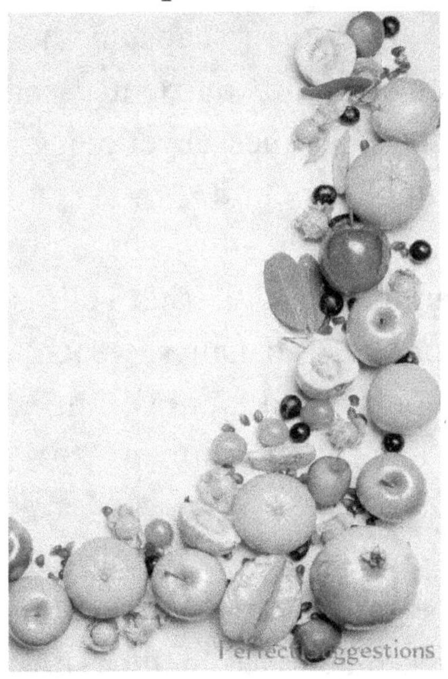

As Quall traveled through her pregnancy, she found the significant job that fruits played in gathering her nourishing necessities and supporting her general prosperity. With each brilliant expansion to her plate, she wound up sustained by the energetic flavors as well as by the abundance of fundamental Vitamins that fruits gave.

One of the most momentous parts of fruits, Quall understood, was their capacity to convey a different cluster of nutrients and minerals fundamental for her wellbeing and the improvement of her child.

From Vitamin c acid rich citrus fruits to potassium-pressed bananas, each Fruit she consumed contributed its novel mix of Vitamins to her everyday eating regimen.

Quall wondered about how fruits easily satisfied her body's requirements for fundamental nutrients and minerals. Whether she was longing for the delicious pleasantness of ready berries or the invigorating smash of fresh apples, she realized that each chomp carried her one bit nearer to meeting her wholesome necessities during pregnancy.

Besides, the fiber content in fruits assumed an urgent part in supporting Quall's stomach related wellbeing and guaranteeing normal solid discharges.

As she enjoyed fiber-rich fruits like kiwi and oranges, she found help from normal inconveniences like clogging, a typical worry during pregnancy.

Hydration was one more part of Quall's pregnancy process that fruits helped address. With their high water content, fruits like watermelon and strawberries gave an invigorating way to Quall to remain hydrated, supporting her body's expanded liquid necessities during pregnancy.

The cell Antioxidantss found richly in fruits offered Quall an additional layer of assurance against oxidative pressure and aggravation, assisting with defending both her and her child's wellbeing. Whether she was appreciating the rich tones of blueberries or the dynamic reds of raspberries, Quall realized that she was supporting her body with strong cell Antioxidantss that advanced ideal wellbeing and prosperity.

As Quall kept on integrating various fruits into her pregnancy diet, she wondered about the significant effect they had on her general wellbeing and imperativeness. Over the long haul, she felt a significant sensation of appreciation for the flood of nature's overflow and the work that natural items played in taking care of her body and supporting her creating youngsters.

Through the sweet flavors and fiery shades of regular items, Quall found food as well as fulfillment and fulfillment in her pregnancy cycle. With each bite, she lauded the superb enrichment of life and the remarkable power of nature's overflow to take care of, recover, and support her through this wondrous piece of being a parent.

Here is a brief summary on how fruits contribute to fulfilling various nutritional needs:

1. Nutrients and Minerals: fruits are loaded with many nutrients and minerals that are fundamental for generally wellbeing. For instance, citrus fruits like oranges and grapefruits are plentiful in Vitamin c acid, which upholds safe capability and skin wellbeing. Bananas are a decent wellspring of potassium, significant for heart wellbeing and muscle capability. Berries like strawberries and blueberries give cancer prevention agents like vitamin E and anthocyanins, which assist with safeguarding cells from harm.

2. Fiber: fruits are an incredible wellspring of dietary fiber, which is significant for stomach related wellbeing and normal defecations. Fiber likewise assists control with blooding sugar levels, lower cholesterol, and advance a sensation of completion, which can support weight on the board. Fiber-rich fruits incorporate apples, pears, berries, and kiwi.

3. Hydration: Many fruits have high water content, which adds to hydration. Remaining hydrated is significant for general wellbeing, as water is engaged with various physical processes, including temperature guideline, Vitamin transport, and waste evacuation. Watermelon, strawberries, and oranges are instances of fruits with high water content.

4. Antioxidants: fruits are wealthy in cancer prevention agents, which assist with safeguarding cells from harm brought about by free revolutionaries. Cell Antioxidantss assume a part in diminishing the gamble of ongoing illnesses like coronary illness, disease, and diabetes. Instances of cell Antioxidants rich fruits incorporate berries, cherries, and grapes.

5. Normal Sugars: While fruits contain regular sugars, they additionally give fundamental Vitamins and fiber, not at all like added sugars tracked down in handled food varieties. The normal sugars in fruits give a fast wellspring of energy, making them a solid choice for fulfilling sweet desires. Matching fruits with protein or solid fats can assist with settling glucose levels and give supported energy.

6. Weight The executives: Remembering fruits for the eating regimen can uphold weight the executives endeavors because of their low calorie thickness and high fiber content. Picking fruits as bites or integrating them into dinners can assist with expanding sensations of totality and fulfillment while lessening by and large calorie intake

Overall, fruits are a Vitamin thick and tasty method for meeting nourishing prerequisites and backing by and large wellbeing. Remembering different fruits for your eating regimen can assist with guaranteeing you get many fundamental nutrients, minerals, fiber, and cell Antioxidantss essential for ideal wellbeing and well-being.

Chapter 3

Safety Guidelines for Consuming Fruits During Pregnancy

As Quall embraced the job of fruits in gathering her nourishing prerequisites during pregnancy, she likewise found out about the significance of consuming them in a protected and adjusted way.

Directed by her medical care supplier and the most recent dietary suggestions, Quall kept a bunch of rules to guarantee she delighted in fruits securely and ideally during this unique time in her life.

1. Wash Completely: Quall regularly practiced it to completely wash all fruits before utilization to eliminate any potential pesticide deposits, soil, or microbes. This straightforward step diminished the gamble of foodborne ailments

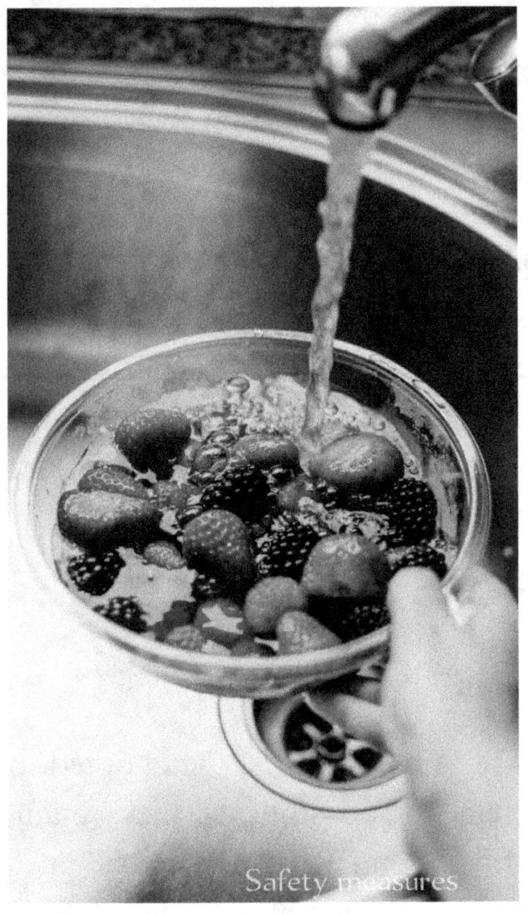

and guaranteed that she and her child remained solid.

2. Choose a Variety: Quall understood the importance of incorporating a variety of fruits into her diet to benefit from a wide range of nutrients. She enjoyed mixing and matching different fruits throughout the week, ensuring she received a diverse array of vitamins, minerals, and antioxidants.

3. Practice Portion Control: While fruits are nutritious, they also contain natural sugars, and consuming them in excess could lead to an imbalance in blood sugar levels. Quall practiced portion control by enjoying fruits as part of balanced meals and snacks, rather than consuming large quantities in one sitting.

4. Include Whole Fruits: Quall opted for whole fruits whenever possible, as they retained their natural fiber content, which aided in digestion and helps regulate blood sugar levels. She enjoyed apples, pears, berries, and other whole fruits as convenient snacks or additions to meals.

5. Be Mindful of Fruit Juices: While fruit juices can be a convenient way to enjoy fruits, Quall was mindful of their high sugar content and low fiber content. She preferred whole fruits over fruit juices whenever possible to maximize fiber intake and minimize sugar spikes.

6. Opt for Fresh or Frozen: Quall prioritized fresh or frozen fruits over canned varieties whenever possible. Fresh and frozen fruits tended to retain more nutrients and had fewer added sugars and preservatives compared to canned fruits.

7. Consider Seasonal Options: Quall embraced seasonal fruits as they not only offered peak flavor and freshness but also tended to be more affordable. She enjoyed exploring farmers' markets and local produce stands to discover seasonal treasures that nourished both her body and soul.

8. Listen to Your Body: Lastly, Quall listened to her body's cues and cravings when it came to consuming fruits. She trusted her instincts and enjoyed fruits that appealed to her taste buds, knowing that her body was intuitively guiding her towards the nutrients she needed during pregnancy.

By keeping these rules, Quall guaranteed that she appreciated fruits securely and dependably all through her pregnancy, receiving the various wellbeing rewards they gave to herself and her developing child.

Organic vs. Conventional Fruits

As Quall navigated her pregnancy journey, she found herself faced with the decision of whether to choose organic or conventional fruits for herself and her growing baby. With growing concerns about pesticides and environmental toxins, Quall sought guidance on the best approach to ensure the safety and healthfulness of the fruits she consumed.

Organic fruits, she learned, were grown without synthetic pesticides, fertilizers, or genetically modified organisms (GMOs).

All things being equal, farmers utilized normal methods like yield revolution, treating the soil, and organic irritation control to support soil wellbeing and shield crops..

Quall valued the accentuation on maintainability and ecological stewardship that natural cultivating rehearses advanced.

Conventional fruits, on the other hand, were typically grown using synthetic pesticides and fertilizers to control pests and enhance crop yields. While conventional farming methods often resulted in larger harvests and lower costs, Quall was concerned about the potential health risks associated with pesticide residues on fruits.

After careful consideration and weighing the pros and cons of each option, Quall decided to prioritize organic fruits whenever possible during her pregnancy. She recognized that while organic fruits might be slightly more expensive and less readily available than conventional fruits, the peace of mind and health benefits they offered were well worth the investment.

By picking normal natural items, Quall restricted her receptiveness to designed pesticides and other disastrous fabricated materials, reducing anticipated risks to herself and her kid. She valued realizing that the fruits she consumed were developed as per severe natural guidelines, liberated from counterfeit added substances and hereditarily adjusted fixings.

Steps in Preparing Fruits Safe

As Quall continued her journey through pregnancy, she recognized the importance of washing and preparing fruits safely to minimize the risk of food borne illnesses and ensure the health and well-being of herself and her growing baby. Armed with knowledge and guidance from her healthcare provider, Quall adopted a series of practices to ensure the safety of the fruits she consumed.

1. Wash Thoroughly: Quall made it a habit to wash all fruits thoroughly before consuming them, regardless of whether they were organic or conventional. She rinsed fruits under cool, running water, gently scrubbing them with a clean brush or cloth to remove any dirt, bacteria, or pesticide residues that may be present on the surface.

2. Handle with Care: Quall handled fruits with care, being mindful not to bruise or damage them during washing or preparation. She avoided washing fruits until just before eating or using them to prevent them from becoming waterlogged and losing their freshness.

3. Peel When Possible: For fruits with thick or tough skins, such as oranges, bananas, and melons, Quall often opted to peel them before consuming them. Peeling fruits removed any potential contaminants on the surface and provided an added layer of protection against bacteria and pesticide residues.

4. Cut Safely: When cutting fruits, Quall used clean utensils and cutting boards to prevent cross-contamination with other foods. She washed her hands thoroughly before and after handling fruits to reduce the risk of transferring harmful bacteria.

5. Store Properly: Quall stored fruits properly to maintain their freshness and minimize the growth of bacteria. She kept fruits in the refrigerator when possible, especially perishable varieties like berries and sliced fruits. Whole fruits like apples and oranges could be stored at room temperature in a cool, dry place away from direct sunlight.

6. Avoid Cross-Contamination: Quall took care to avoid cross-contamination between fruits and other foods in the kitchen. She kept fruits separate from raw meat, poultry, seafood, and eggs to prevent the spread of harmful bacteria.

7. Consume Promptly: To ensure the highest quality and safety of fruits, Quall consumed them promptly after washing and preparation. She avoided letting cut fruits sit at room temperature for extended periods and refrigerated any leftovers promptly to prevent spoilage.

Quall took proactive measures to safeguard her health and the health of her baby during pregnancy. She found peace of mind in knowing that each delicious bite of fruit she enjoyed was not only nourishing her body but also supporting her journey through this extraordinary chapter of motherhood.

Chapter 4

Best Fruits for Pregnancy and Benefits of Each Fruit for Pregnant Women

1. 0ranges: Oranges are plentiful in Vitamin c acid, which upholds safe capability and collagen creation. They likewise give folate, potassium, and fiber. The high water content of oranges helps keep the body hydrated and helps absorption, going with them a brilliant decision for pregnant ladies.

2. Bananas: Bananas are an incredible wellspring of potassium, which directs pulse and muscle capability. They in like manner give vitamin B6, which is critical for emotional well-being in the youngsterBananas are not difficult to process and can assist with mitigating queasiness and morning infection during pregnancy.

3. Berries (Strawberries, Blueberries, Raspberries): Berries are packed with antioxidants, including vitamin C and flavonoids, which help protect cells from damage. They also provide fiber, which supports digestive health and helps control blood sugar levels. Berries are low in calories and can satisfy sweet cravings in a healthy way.

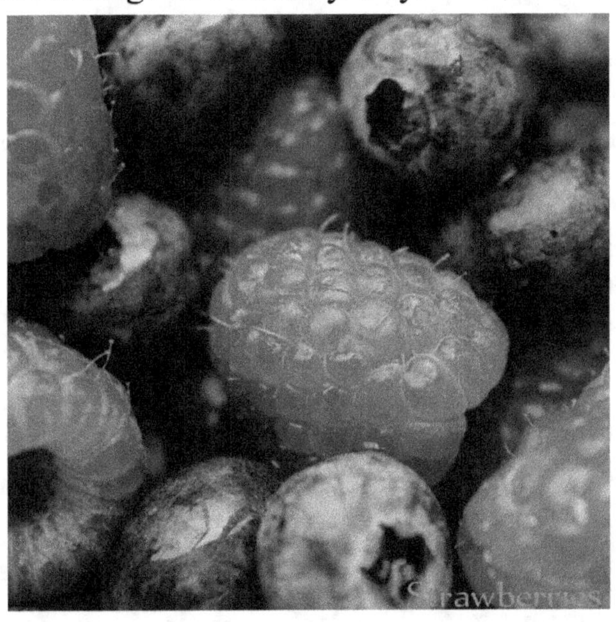

4. Goji berries: Goji berries are high in vitamin A, iron, and cell Antioxidants.
Hemoglobin a protein in red platelets that transports oxygen to the child's tissues and lowers the risk of iron deficiency in the mother, depends on iron for its production.

Antioxidants help to safeguard the kid's tissues and lessen oxidative strain.

5. Acai berries: Acai berries are notable for their high grouping of malignant growth-battling mixtures and fundamental unsaturated fats.
Omega-3 and Omega-6 Unsaturated fats are significant for the advancement of the kid's mind and eyes. They provide healthy support for the mother's cardiovascular health.
Antioxidants help protect the mother's and child's cells from injury.

6. Pomegranates: Pomegranates are recognized for their high levels of cancer-fighting chemicals, vitamins C and K, and folate.
Folate is essential for the proper development of the child's brain tube, which subsequently matures into the cerebrum and spinal cord, lowering the risk of brain tube absconding.
Antioxidants strengthen the immune system and contribute to a healthy bloodstream, promoting overall fetal growth and motherly well-being.

7. Apples: Apples are rich in fiber, vitamin C, and various antioxidants. The soluble fiber in apples helps regulate bowel movements and may reduce the risk of gestational diabetes. Consuming apples with the skin intact offers extra nutrients and fiber

8. Kiwi: Kiwi is loaded with vitamin C, vitamin K, vitamin E, and folate. It also contains digestive enzymes that aid in digestion and promote gut health. The high fiber content of kiwi helps prevent constipation, a common issue during pregnancy

9. Avocado: Avocado is a nutrient-dense fruit that provides healthy fats, including monounsaturated fats and omega-3 fatty acids. It also contains potassium, vitamin K, vitamin E, and folate. Avocado supports fetal brain development and helps regulate blood pressure

10. Papaya: Papaya is rich in vitamins A and C, as well as enzymes like papain and chymopapain, which aid digestion. However, pregnant women should consume papaya in moderation and avoid unripe or semi-ripe papaya, as it contains latex that may stimulate contraction

11. Mango: Mangoes are packed with vitamin C, vitamin A, and folate. They also contain enzymes like amylases and proteases, which aid in digestion. Mangoes are refreshing and can help alleviate cravings for sweet

12. Grapes: Grapes are rich in antioxidants, including resveratrol, which has been linked to heart health and reduced inflammation. They also provide vitamin C, vitamin K, and potassium. Grapes are a convenient and hydrating snack option for pregnant women

13. Pineapple: Pineapple contains bromelain, a compound that might assist with lessening aggravation and further develop absorption. Be that as it may, pregnant ladies ought to consume pineapple with some restraint and try not to eat it in enormous sums, particularly in early pregnancy, as bromelain may cause uterine constriction

Each of these nutrient-rich fruits offers unique benefits for pregnant women, supporting their overall health and the development of their babies.
By adding variety of fruits into their diet, pregnant women can ensure they receive a wide range of essential nutrients to support a healthy pregnancy and childbirth

Chapter 5

Incorporating Fruits into Pregnancy Meal Plans

As Quall proceeded with her pregnancy process, she embraced the significance of integrating various Vitamin rich fruits into her day to day feast intended to help her wellbeing and the advancement of her child. With inventiveness and aim, she tracked down heavenly ways of getting a charge out of fruits over the course of the day, guaranteeing she got a different exhibit of nutrients, minerals, and cell Antioxidantss.

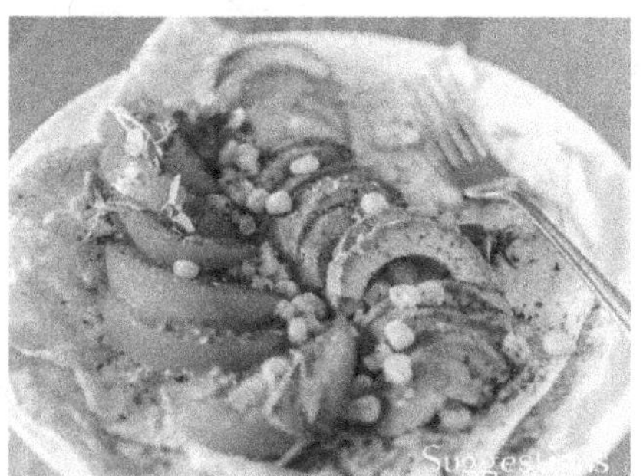

Breakfast

For breakfast, Quall frequently began her day with an invigorating Fruit smoothie. She mixed together fruits, like bananas, berries, and spinach, alongside Greek yogurt and a sprinkle of almond milk. This Vitamin stuffed smoothie gave her an eruption of energy and hydration to launch her morning.

Snacks Options
At mid-morning, Quall enjoyed a snack of sliced apples paired with almond butter or a handful of grapes and nuts.

These straightforward yet fulfilling snacks furnished her with an equilibrium of sugars, protein, and solid fats to keep her powered until noon.

Lunch
For lunch, Quall got innovative with plates of mixed greens highlighting different foods grown from the ground.

She tossed together leafy greens with sliced strawberries, avocado, and grilled chicken, drizzled with a tangy balsamic vinaigrette. Or she enjoyed a tropical-inspired salad with mixed greens, mango, pineapple, and grilled shrimp, topped with a citrusy dressing.

SUPPER
For supper, Quall integrated fruits into appetizing dishes to add flavor and sustenance

She enjoyed grilled salmon with a side of roasted sweet potatoes and steamed broccoli, or she made a colorful stir-fry with chicken, bell peppers, snap peas, and pineapple served over brown rice.

Quall also treated herself to a small bowl of mixed fruit salad, featuring her favorite seasonal fruits like kiwi, grapes and oranges. This light and reviving pastry gave a sweet consummation of her day without burdening her before sleep time.

Throughout her pregnancy, Quall found joy and nourishment in incorporating fruits into her meal plans in creative and satisfying ways.

By focusing on a different exhibit of fruits, she guaranteed she got the fundamental Vitamins expected to help her wellbeing and the development of her child, making every dinner a festival of life and overflow.

Chapter 6

Cultural Perspectives on Fruits and Pregnancy

Traditional Practices

Across various societies, conventional works on Fruits during pregnancy are well established in authentic convictions and the characteristic qualities put on maternal and fetal wellbeing.

These practices frequently underline the regular properties of leafy foods of representative importance, reflecting hundreds of years of gathered astuteness.

1. India

Bananas: In India, bananas are consumed to help process and give energy, which is imperative for hopeful moms encountering a morning ailment or weakness. Bananas are likewise a staple in ceremonies and contributions, mirroring their social significance.

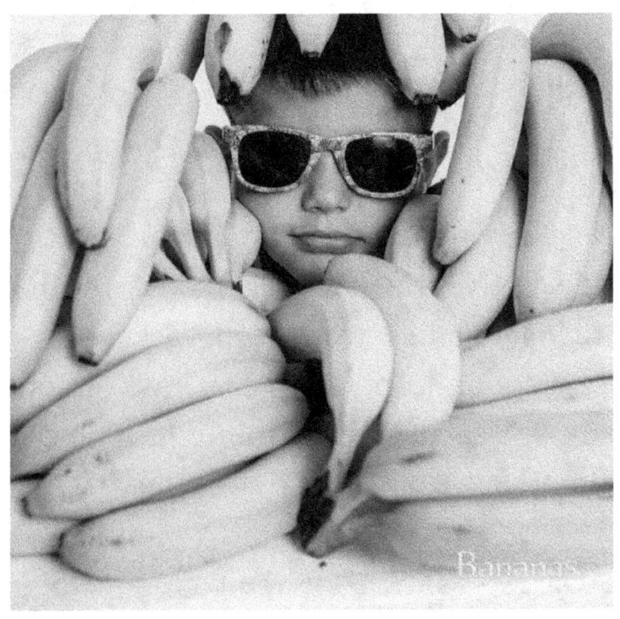

Mangoes: Considered the "ruler of Fruits," mangoes are generally eaten for their rich vitamin A substance, supporting the child's turn of events and the mother's general wellbeing. They are additionally utilized in services, representing richness and flourishing.

Pomegranates: Consumed for their alleged blood-upgrading properties, pomegranates are believed to work on iron levels and support sound blood flow. This training is built up by the

Fruit's noticeable job in customary cures and Ayurvedic medication.

2. China

Pears: Pears are eaten to adjust your energy and cool the body, which is accepted to be helpful for pregnant ladies who need to keep up with their inner amicability. Pears are frequently stewed or eaten fresh to reduce heat and hydration.

Red Dates: Known for their blood-supporting properties, red dates are ordinarily remembered for soups and teas to reinforce the mother's blood and improve general imperativeness. This lines up with the confidence in conventional Chinese medicine that they sustain the body and advance a solid fetal turn of events.

3. Center East

Dates: Dates are generally consumed for their nourishing thickness and energy-giving properties. They are especially esteemed for their part in facilitating work torments, with the conviction that their normal sugars and Vitamins support strength and perseverance during labor.

Figs: Figs are remembered for pregnancy slims down for their high fiber content, helping processing, and forestalling blockage. They are frequently connected with wellbeing and essentialness, representing life span and ripeness.

4. Africa

Baobab Fruit: The baobab Fruit, plentiful in Vitamin c acid and calcium, is generally used to help maternal resistance and reinforce bones. It is often consumed as a powder blended into beverages or porridge.

Tamarind: Tamarind is utilized to battle morning infections because of its tart taste, which decreases queasiness. It is additionally integrated into sauces and beverages to provide fundamental nutrients and minerals.

5. Latin America

Avocados: Avocados are praised for their solid fats and folate content, which are accepted to help mental health and, in general, fetal wellbeing. Customarily, they are integrated into day-to-day dinners like plates of mixed greens and guacamole.

Papayas: In numerous Latin American societies, ready papayas are consumed for their stomach-related benefits, while unripe papayas are kept away because of worries about expected uterine withdrawals.

6. Europe

Figs and Grapes: In Mediterranean societies, figs and grapes are esteemed for their Vitamin thickness and are remembered for pregnancy diets to provide fundamental nutrients and minerals. These Fruits are likewise connected to social practices that underline new, occasional produce.

Berries: In Northern Europe, berries like blueberries and lingonberries are consumed for their high Vitamin c acid and cell Antioxidants content, supporting resistant capability and fetal turn of events.

7. Native Societies

Cranberries and Wild Berries: Local American practices use cranberries and wild berries for their restorative properties, supporting maternal wellbeing and preventing urinary tract contamination and different infirmities.

Feijoa and Kiwi: In Maori culture, feijoa and kiwi are integrated into the eating regimen for their high Vitamin c acid and folate content, supporting maternal wellbeing and fetal turn of events.

Worldwide Dietary Examples

In contemporary nourishment, there is a developing appreciation for the customary utilization of Fruits in pregnancy calorie counts.

These worldwide dietary examples incorporate conventional insight with current nourishing science, underscoring the different advantages of Fruits for hopeful moms.

1. Accentuation on Vitamin Thickness

Current dietary examples focus on Fruits that offer high Vitamin thickness, lining up with conventional practices that value Fruits for their particular medical advantages. This remembers a concentration for:

Cell Antioxidantss: Fruits like berries, rich in cancer prevention agents, are consumed to safeguard cells and advance solid turns of events.

Nutrients and Minerals: Citrus leafy foods Fruits are esteemed for their Vitamin c acid and folate content, supporting invulnerable capability and fetal development.

2. Joining of Super Fruits

The worldwide acknowledgment of super Fruits like açai, goji berries, and pomegranates mirrors a mix of conventional and present-day dietary examples. These Fruits are praised for their remarkable Vitamin profiles and their capacity to improve maternal and fetal wellbeing.

3. Occasional and neighborhood eating

Many societies underscore the utilization of occasional and privately developed Fruits, a training that lines up with present-day suggestions for new, Vitamin-rich produce. This approach upholds supportable eating practices and gives the freshest and most nutritious choices that anyone could hope to find.

4. Utilitarian food sources

There is a rising pattern towards utilitarian food sources, which are food varieties that offer medical advantages beyond essential sustenance. Fruits that help explicit wellbeing capabilities, for example, stomach-related wellbeing or glucose guidelines, are becoming fundamental to pregnancy eats less carbs around the world.

5. All-encompassing well-being

Worldwide dietary examples are progressively all-encompassing, perceiving the interconnectedness of physical, mental, and profound wellbeing. Fruits are incorporated for their actual advantages as well as for their part in advancing general prosperity and essentialness during pregnancy.

Conclusion

The coordination of customary practices and current worldwide dietary examples highlights the general worth of Fruits in supporting a solid pregnancy.

By embracing both verifiable insight and contemporary, nourishing bits of knowledge, hopeful moms can partake in a reasonable eating regimen that advances the prosperity of both mother and child.

Chapter 7

Addressing Common Concerns

As Quall navigated her pregnancy journey, she encountered some common concerns about fruit consumption that echoed among expectant mothers.

While she embraced the importance of incorporating fruits into her diet for their nutritional benefits, she also remained mindful of potential concerns and took proactive steps to address them.

One of the primary concerns among pregnant women was the presence of pesticide residues on fruits, especially those conventionally grown. Quall understood the importance of minimizing exposure to pesticides during pregnancy and chose to prioritize organic fruits whenever possible. By opting for organic varieties or fruits with thicker skins that could be peeled, she felt reassured that she was reducing potential risks to herself and her baby.

Foodborne illnesses were another concern that weighed heavily on Quall's mind. With her immune system changing during pregnancy, she was aware of the heightened risk of foodborne illnesses and the importance of safe food handling practices.

Quall made it a priority to wash fruits thoroughly before consumption and followed guidelines for storing and preparing fruits safely to minimize the risk of contamination.

As she learned more about gestational diabetes and its implications for pregnancy, Quall became mindful of the sugar content of fruits and its impact on blood sugar levels. While she enjoyed the natural sweetness of fruits, she was cautious about consuming them in excess and opted for lower-sugar varieties when possible. Quall worked closely with her healthcare provider to manage her blood sugar levels while including fruits in her meal plans in moderation.

Being aware of potential allergies was also essential for Quall as she considered her fruit choices during pregnancy.

While she didn't have any known allergies herself, she took precautions to avoid fruits that could potentially trigger allergic reactions in herself or her unborn baby.

Quall remained vigilant about reading food labels and monitoring her body's responses to different fruits to ensure a safe and healthy pregnancy.

Ultimately, Quall was aware of what certain fruits could mean for her gastrointestinal wellbeing during pregnancy. As she experienced occasional bouts of heartburn and indigestion, she learned to choose fruits that were less acidic and less likely to exacerbate these symptoms.

She likewise made a point to incorporate high-fiber fruits in her eating regimen to assist with lightning obstruction, a typical worry among pregnant ladies

Here are more testimonies from pregnant womens who utilized the power of fruits.

Emma's Story:
Overseeing Pre-birth Diabetes with Apples

Emma's pregnancy was met with happiness and energy, yet additionally with a critical test that additional a layer of intricacy to her excursion: pre-birth diabetes.

Analyzed during her subsequent trimester, Emma was educated that she would have to painstakingly screen her glucose levels and stick to a severe eating regimen to guarantee the wellbeing and security of both herself and her creating child.

The finding came as a shock. Emma had consistently viewed herself as somewhat solid and dynamic, and the news that she had gestational diabetes filled her with nervousness and vulnerability.

She was very much in the know about the dangers related with uncontrolled glucose levels during pregnancy, including preterm birth, unreasonable birth weight, and the potential for creating type 2 diabetes further down the road.

Not set in stone to deal with her condition successfully, Emma dove into research, searching out food sources that would assist with directing her glucose levels while as yet giving the vital Vitamins to her and her child.

It was during this search that she ran over the modest apple, a Fruit she had consistently delighted in however never viewed as a basic piece of her eating routine.

Emma discovered that apples, especially when eaten with their skins, are high in dietary fiber, which eases back the assimilation of sugar into the circulatory system.

This property pursued them an optimal decision for dealing with her glucose levels. She chose to integrate apples into her day to day daily schedule, eating them as snacks among dinners and adding them to her plates of mixed greens and breakfast dishes.

To her enjoyment, Emma observed that apples were not just powerful in assisting her with dealing with her glucose levels, however they likewise gave a large group of different advantages.

Their high fiber content kept her feeling full and energized throughout the day, and their natural sweetness satisfied her cravings without raising her blood sugar. She could partake in a heavenly, fulfilling tidbit that upheld her wellbeing objectives, which was a huge help given her dietary limitations.

Emma began her mornings with a bowl of oats finished off with cut apples and a sprinkle of cinnamon, a mix that turned into her number one method for beginning the day.

For lunch, she frequently remembered a green apple for her serving of mixed greens, adding a reviving crunch and an explosion of flavor. She found that an apple was the perfect pick-me-up in the afternoons, when she usually had less energy, and that it didn't upset her blood sugar like sugary snacks did.

Through cautious observing and predictable dietary changes, Emma had the option to keep her glucose levels inside the suggested range. Her commitment to dealing with her eating routine paid off, and she effectively conveyed her pregnancy to term without difficulties connected with her gestational diabetes.

Emma's experience highlights the strong effect that straightforward, normal food varieties can have on overseeing medical issues during pregnancy. Her revelation of the advantages of apples not just assisted her with exploring the difficulties of pre-birth diabetes yet in addition enhanced how she might interpret sustenance and health.

By embracing the force of fruits, she figured out how to help her wellbeing and the strength of her child in a scrumptious and supportable way.

Sarah's Story:
Finding Solace in Watermelon
Sarah had a lot of joy and excitement as she prepared to become a mother, but she also had terrible morning sickness, a problem that many aspiring moms are all too acquainted with. From the beginning of her most memorable trimester,

Sarah was struck with waves of nausea that seemed to never end.

The medical term for the illness is hyperemesis gravidarum, which left her feeling depressed and hopeless, unable to eat a large meal, and always anxious for her child's health. No significant lightning was obtained with conventional procedures.

She sought relief, but ginger tea, wafers, and prescription medications from the doctor didn't cut it. She may have nausea at any time of day, not only in the morning, which makes it difficult for her to work, socialize, or even get a good night's sleep.

She came to terms with the fact that she was caught in a never-ending cycle of disease and exhaustion and that her struggle to survive was more important than her happiness.

One especially sweltering evening, after an especially unpleasant morning, Sarah's companion visited her with a huge, delicious watermelon. Sarah was initially skeptical—how could a straightforward fruit help when so many other treatments had failed? However, she was open to trying anything. She cut into the watermelon, its dazzling red tissue and invigorating fragrance offering a good omen.

Taking her most memorable nibble, Sarah was agreeably amazed by the unobtrusive causticity of the Fruit. The delicate corrosiveness was calming on her stomach, in contrast to the more keen preferences that frequently exacerbated her queasiness.

As she kept on eating, she found that the cooling kind of the watermelon appeared to quiet her agitated stomach. Something other than lightening her sickness, the high water content of the watermelon helped keep her hydrated, a basic component given how frequently she had been not able to hold liquids down.

Watermelon turned into a staple in Sarah's eating routine. She kept cuts of it in the cooler, prepared to snatch at whatever point she felt the sickness crawling back.

It was not difficult to process, gave an invigorating explosion of hydration, and assisted her with keeping up with her solidarity through those troublesome first months.

Over the long run, as her queasiness died down, Sarah began to explore different avenues regarding different fruits, yet she generally kept watermelon nearby as she confided in its cure.

Sarah's experience is an exhibition of the direct yet massive impact that the right food can have during pregnancy. Her story isn't just about finding help from a regular pregnancy illness, yet about tracking down a trademark and strong strategy for supporting her success. She learned how to trust the delicate force of nature's contributions during her trip, which was an example that guided her through the remainder of her pregnancy with confidence and beauty.

Managing Gestational Diabetes with Fruits

Gestational diabetes mellitus (GDM) is a type of diabetes that can develop during pregnancy. It is characterized by elevated blood sugar levels that begin or are first detected during this period. Managing gestational diabetes is crucial to ensure the health and well-being of both the mother and the baby.

When it comes to managing gestational diabetes, including fruits in the diet can be a healthy and nutritious choice. However, pregnant women with gestational diabetes need to be mindful of their fruit intake and its impact on blood sugar levels.

Here are some tips for managing gestational diabetes with fruits:

1.   Choose   Low-Glycemic   Fruits: Low-glycemic fruits have a lower impact on blood sugar levels compared to high-glycemic fruits. Examples of low-glycemic fruits include berries (such as strawberries, blueberries, and raspberries), cherries, and apples. These fruits are less likely to cause rapid spikes in blood sugar levels and can be included in moderation in the diet of women with gestational diabetes.

2. Portion Control: While fruits are nutritious, they contain natural sugars that can still affect blood sugar levels. Pregnant women with gestational diabetes should practice portion control when consuming fruits. It's essential to be mindful of portion sizes and not to overindulge, even with low-glycemic fruits.

3. Pair with Protein or Healthy Fats: Pairing fruits with protein or healthy fats can help slow down the absorption of sugars into the bloodstream and minimize the impact on blood sugar levels. For example, pregnant women can enjoy sliced apples with almond butter or Greek yogurt with berries for a balanced snack.

4. Monitor Blood Sugar Levels: Pregnant women with gestational diabetes should monitor their blood sugar levels regularly as advised by their healthcare provider. Keeping track of blood sugar levels can help identify any spikes or fluctuations and guide adjustments to the diet and lifestyle as needed.

5. Spread Fruit Consumption Throughout the Day: Rather than consuming all fruits at once, pregnant women with gestational diabetes can spread their fruit consumption throughout the day. This can help prevent rapid increases in blood sugar levels and promote better blood sugar control.

6. Include High-Fiber Fruits: High-fiber fruits can help regulate blood sugar levels and promote satiety, making them beneficial for managing gestational diabetes. Examples of high-fiber fruits include pears, oranges, and kiwi. Including these fruits in the diet can help support digestive health and blood sugar management.

7. Talk with an Enlisted Dietitian: Pregnant ladies with gestational diabetes ought to work intimately with an enlisted dietitian or medical services supplier to foster a customized dinner plan that meets their dietary necessities and oversees glucose levels. A dietitian can give direction on integrating fruits into the eating regimen such that upholds ideal wellbeing during pregnancy.

By following these tips and working closely with their healthcare team, pregnant women with gestational diabetes can effectively manage their condition while still enjoying the health benefits of fruits as part of a balanced die

Conclusion

As Quall's pregnancy process came to a close, she pondered the endless manners by which fruits had improved her experience and upheld her wellbeing all through this striking time. From the early stages of conception to the final days of anticipation, fruits had been a constant source of nourishment, vitality, and joy for Quall and her growing baby.

The benefits of incorporating fruits into her pregnancy diet were abundant and undeniable:

1. Essential Nutrients: Fruits provided a wide range of essential vitamins, minerals, and antioxidants that supported Quall's overall health and the development of her baby. From vitamin C to folate to potassium, each fruit offered a unique blend of nutrients crucial for a healthy pregnancy.

2. Hydration: With their high water content, fruits helped keep Quall hydrated, especially during moments when drinking plain water felt challenging. Whether she savored juicy watermelon slices or enjoyed a refreshing berry smoothie, fruits provided a delicious and hydrating option for staying nourished and refreshed.

3. Digestive Health: The fiber found in fruits played a vital role in promoting healthy digestion and regular bowel movements for Quall. As she navigated the occasional discomforts of pregnancy, such as constipation and bloating, fruits provided natural relief and support for her digestive system.

4. Immune Boosting: The vitamins and antioxidants in fruits bolstered Quall's immune system, helping her stay strong and resilient throughout her pregnancy. From fighting off common colds to protecting against infections, fruits served as a powerful ally in maintaining her health and well-being.

5. Gestational Diabetes Management: Quall learned how to incorporate fruits into her pregnancy diet in a way that supported healthy blood sugar levels, even managing gestational diabetes with careful attention to portion sizes and choosing low-glycemic fruits. By working intimately with her medical services supplier and pursuing informed decisions, she found equilibrium and strength in her glucose levels while as yet partaking in the advantages of fruits.

6. Morning Disorder Help: Certain fruits, like ginger and citrus, gave normal alleviation to Quall's morning ailment side effects. Whether she sipped on ginger tea or indulged in a slice of fresh orange, fruits offered comfort and soothing relief during moments of nausea and discomfort.

7. Overall Well-Being: Beyond their nutritional benefits, fruits brought a sense of joy, vibrancy, and connection to Quall's pregnancy journey.

From the bright cluster of fruits at the ranchers' market to the common snapshots of satisfaction with friends and family, fruits turned out to be something other than food — they turned into an image of life, love, and overflow

As Quall arranged to invite her little one into the world, she conveyed with her a profound appreciation for the job that fruits had played in supporting her through this mind blowing venture

With each bite of fruit, she celebrated the miracle of life and the profound connection she shared with her baby, knowing that she had provided them with the best possible start in life through the power of fruits and wholesome nutrition

As she anticipated the undertakings that lay ahead, Quall realized that the examples she had learned and the recollections she had made during her pregnancy would remain with her eternity, filling in as a sign of the unlimited love and vast conceivable outcomes that looked for her and her developing family.

So as you close this book, remember that the journey of pregnancy is enriched by the natural gifts of fruits. Each vibrant piece not only nourishes your body but also supports the growth and well-being of your baby. Embrace the bounty of nature, and let every bite be a step toward a healthier, happier future for both you and your child. Here's to the sweet journey of motherhood, nourished by nature's finest offerings."

- Final Tips for a Healthy Pregnancy Journey

1. Prioritize Nutrition: Focus on consuming a balanced diet rich in fruits, vegetables, lean proteins, whole grains, and healthy fats to support your health and the development of your baby. Aim to eat a variety of nutrient-dense foods and stay hydrated throughout the day.

2. Stay Active: Incorporate regular physical activity into your routine, as long as it's approved by your healthcare provider. Engaging in activities such as walking, swimming, and prenatal yoga can enhance circulation, alleviate stress, and ready your body for childbirth.

3. Get Plenty of Rest: Listen to your body's cues and prioritize rest and relaxation. Aim for 7-9 hours of quality sleep each night and take breaks throughout the day to recharge. Proper rest is essential for your physical and emotional well-being during pregnancy.

4. Stay Hydrated: Drink plenty of water throughout the day to stay hydrated and support your body's needs. Aim for at least 8-10 glasses of water per day, and adjust your intake as needed based on factors like activity level and climate.

5. Attend Prenatal Appointments: Keep up with regular prenatal check-ups and appointments with your healthcare provider. These visits are essential for monitoring your health, tracking your baby's growth and development, and addressing any concerns or questions you may have.

6. Educate Yourself: Take the time to learn about pregnancy, childbirth, and newborn care through books, classes, and reputable online resources. Knowledge is empowering, and being informed can help you make confident decisions throughout your pregnancy journey.

7. Practice Self-Care: Make self-care a priority by engaging in activities that bring you joy and relaxation. Whether it's taking a warm bath, practicing mindfulness meditation, or indulging in a prenatal massage, find ways to nurture your body and mind during pregnancy.

8. Connect with Supportive Community: Surround yourself with a supportive network of family, friends, and healthcare professionals who can offer guidance, encouragement, and reassurance during your pregnancy journey. Joining a prenatal support group or online community can also provide valuable support and camaraderie.

9. Prepare for Birth: Educate yourself about the birthing process and explore your options for childbirth, including pain management techniques, labor positions, and birthing preferences. Consider creating a birth plan that outlines your preferences and priorities for labor and delivery.

10. Trust Your Instincts: Finally, trust your instincts and intuition as you navigate through pregnancy and prepare for motherhood. Listen to your body, advocate for your needs, and trust in your ability to make the best decisions for yourself and your baby.

By following these tips and embracing the journey with an open heart and mind, you can enjoy a healthy and fulfilling pregnancy experience, laying the foundation for a lifetime of love and joy with your little one.

Appendix

Nutritional chart

Understanding the wholesome substance of different Fruits is critical for making a reasonable pregnancy diet. This graph gives nitty-gritty data on fundamental Vitamins tracked down in ordinarily suggested Fruits for pregnant ladies.

Fruits	Calories	Vitamin c (mg)	Folate (mcg)	Fiber (g)	Potassium (mg)	Iron (mg)	ioxidants (ORAC)
Apple	95	8	5	4	195	0.2	2,983
Bananas	105	10	24	3	42	0.3	795
Blueberry	84	14	9	4	114	0.4	4,669
Mango	99	60	71	3	277	0.2	1,005
Avocado	234	15	89	10	708	0.8	1,933
Orange	62	70	30	3	237	0.1	2,103
Pomegranate	234	28	38	11	666	0.5	4,479
[illegible]	43	[illegible]	19	[illegible]	[illegible]	[illegible]	[illegible]
Grape	62	4	3	1	176	0.5	1,837
Strawberry	49	89	35	3	233	0.4	4,302
[illegible]	282	0.4	15	6	656	0.9	3,895
[illegible]	82	79	40	3	190	0.3	1,429

ORAC (Oxygen Extremist Absorbance Limit) measures cancer prevention agent levels.

Suggested Everyday Admission

Guaranteeing sufficient admission of fundamental Vitamins during pregnancy upholds both maternal wellbeing and the fetal turn of events. This part gives rules for the day-to-day admission of basic nutrients and minerals, along with ideas on how Fruits can contribute to meeting these necessities.

1. Vitamin

Vitamin: 85 mg/day
Role: Keeps up with the safeguarded framework, maintains iron processing, and advances solid skin.
Sources: oranges (70 mg for every medium-normal thing), strawberries (89 mg for each cup), and kiwis (71 mg for every regular thing).
Vitamin A: 770 mcg/day
Role: Fundamental for fetal turn of events, vision, and safe capacity.
Sources: mangoes (112 mcg for each cup), papayas (95 mcg for each cup).

Folate (vitamin B9): 600 mcg/day
Role: Fundamental for DNA blend and the improvement of the brain tube.
Sources: avocados (89 mcg for every natural item), oranges (30 mcg for each medium-normal item).

2. Minerals

Iron (27 mg/day)
Role: maintains the making of hemoglobin and thwarts shortcoming.
Sources: pomegranates (0.5 mg per natural item) and dates (0.9 mg per 100 g).

Calcium: 1,000 mg/day.
Role: Huge to improve the kid's bones and teeth.
Sources: oranges (52 mg for each medium natural item), figs (90 mg for each 100 g dried).

Potassium: 2,900–3,500 mg/day
Role: Stays aware of fluid harmony, maintains nerve ability, and prevents muscle cramps.

Sources: bananas (422 mg for each medium-regular thing), avocados (708 mg for every normal thing).

3. Fiber

Fiber: 28 g/day
Role: It helps with absorption and prevent constipation.
Sources: apples (4 g for each medium regular thing), blueberries (4 g for each cup).

Glossary of Terms

Antioxidants

Intensifies that safeguard the body's cells from harm brought about by free extremists, which are temperamental particles that can prompt oxidative pressure and add to persistent sicknesses. Normal cell Antioxidantss found in Fruits incorporate Vitamin c, vitamin E, and polyphenols.

Dietary Fiber

A kind of starch found in plant food sources that isn't processed by the human body. Fiber helps with keeping up with stomach-related wellbeing, controlling glucose levels, and bringing down cholesterol. Fruits like apples, berries, and pears are high in fiber.

Folate (Vitamin B9)

A water-solvent nutrient is vital for DNA union, cell development, and the legitimate improvement of the brain tube in babies. Folate is especially important during pregnancy to prevent brain tube depletion. It is plentiful in avocados, oranges, and verdant green vegetables.

Iron

A mineral fundamental for making hemoglobin, the protein in red platelets that conveys oxygen all through the body. During pregnancy, iron necessities increase to help the developing hatchling and placenta. Dates and pomegranates are added to iron-rich Fruits.

Omega-3 and Omega-6 Unsaturated Fats

Fundamental unsaturated fats that assume an imperative role in cerebrum capability, typical development and improvement, and irritation guidelines These are regularly tracked down in greasy fish, yet they are also present in certain Fruits like açai berries.

ORAC (Oxygen Radical Absorbance Capacity)
A strategy for estimating the cell antioxidant limit of various food varieties. Fruits with high ORAC values, like blueberries and

pomegranates, are viewed as powerful in killing free revolutionaries.

Potassium

A mineral that manages liquid equilibrium, muscle constrictions, and nerve signals. Satisfactory potassium admission can assist with forestalling muscle squeezes and keeping up with solid circulatory strain. Bananas and avocados are brilliant wellsprings of potassium.

Super Fruits

Fruits that are uncommonly wealthy in Vitamins and cancer prevention agents offer critical medical advantages. Models incorporate blueberries, pomegranates, and açai berries, known for their elevated degrees of nutrients, minerals, and phytonutrients.

Vitamin c

A water-dissolvable nutrient is fundamental for the development and fixation of tissues in the body, the development of collagen, and the retention of iron from plant-based food varieties. Vitamin c acid is abundant in citrus Fruits, strawberries, and kiwis.

Vitamin E

A fat-solvent cell antioxidants that safeguards cells from oxidative harm and supports invulnerable capability. It is found in limited quantities in many Fruits, particularly berries.

Conclusion

This index gives a far-reaching outline of fundamental healthful data for Fruits ordinarily suggested during pregnancy. By grasping the nourishing substance, suggested everyday admission, and key terms connected with pregnancy sustenance, eager moms can pursue informed decisions to help their wellbeing and the advancement of their child.

References

Studies and Articles on Pregnancy Nutrition Understanding the impact of nutrition during pregnancy is crucial for promoting maternal and fetal health. Here are some key studies and articles that provide valuable insights into the role of fruits and other nutrients during pregnancy:

1. "Nutritional Needs During Pregnancy" by the American College of Obstetricians and Gynecologists (ACOG)
   - This comprehensive guide outlines the essential vitamins and minerals required during pregnancy and emphasizes the importance of a balanced diet including fruits.
   - Available at: [ACOG](https://www.acog.org)

2. "The Role of Antioxidants in Pregnancy" by the Journal of Nutritional Biochemistry

- This study explores how antioxidants from fruits like berries and pomegranates can protect maternal and fetal cells from oxidative stress.
   - DOI: 10.1016/j.jnutbio.2019.03.007

3. "Impact of Maternal Nutrition on Fetal Development" by the World Health Organization (WHO)
   - This report discusses how maternal nutrition, including fruit intake, influences fetal development and long-term health outcomes.
   - Available at: [WHO](https://www.who.int)

4. "Fruit Consumption During Pregnancy and Its Effects on Birth Outcomes" by the American Journal of Clinical Nutrition
   - This article reviews various studies on the positive effects of fruit consumption on birth weight, gestational age, and overall neonatal health.
   - DOI: 10.1093/ajcn/nqz245

5. "Folate and Pregnancy: A Review of the Evidence" by the National Institutes of Health (NIH)

   - This review highlights the critical role of folate in preventing neural tube defects and discusses dietary sources including fruits.

   - Available at: [NIH](https://www.nih.gov)

Further Reading and Resources

For those looking to deepen their understanding of pregnancy nutrition, these books, websites, and organizations offer extensive information and practical advice:

1. Books

   - "What to Eat When You're Pregnant" by Nicole M. Avena, Ph.D.

   - This book provides detailed guidance on the best foods to eat during pregnancy, including the benefits of various fruits.

- "The Whole 9 Months: A Week-by-Week Pregnancy Nutrition Guide with Recipes for a Healthy Start" by Jennifer Lang, MD
    - A comprehensive guide that offers weekly nutritional advice and recipes to support a healthy pregnancy.

- "Expecting Better: Why the Conventional Pregnancy Wisdom Is Wrong—and What You Really Need to Know" by Emily Oster
    - This book challenges traditional pregnancy advice with data-driven insights, including nutritional guidelines.

2. Websites

- Mayo Clinic Pregnancy Nutrition
    - Offers expert advice on nutritional needs during pregnancy, including recommended fruit intake.
    - Available at: [Mayo Clinic](https://www.mayoclinic.org)

- March of Dimes

- Provides information on pregnancy health, including nutrition tips and the benefits of fruit consumption.
   - Available at: [March of Dimes](https://www.marchofdimes.org)

- Healthy Eating During Pregnancy by the U.S. Department of Health and Human Services (HHS)
   - Detailed guidelines on maintaining a balanced diet during pregnancy.
   - Available at: [HHS](https://www.hhs.gov)

3. Organizations and Resources

- American Pregnancy Association (APA)
   - A non-profit organization offering educational materials on pregnancy nutrition and health.
   - Available at: [American Pregnancy](https://americanpregnancy.org)

- World Health Organization (WHO) - Nutrition in Pregnancy

- Provides global guidelines and resources on nutrition for expectant mothers.
   - Available at: [WHO](https://www.who.int)

   - National Institutes of Health (NIH) - Pregnancy Nutrition
   - Offers a wealth of research and information on dietary needs during pregnancy.
   - Available at: [NIH](https://www.nih.gov)